Juicing for   s Syndrome

How I Treated My RLS by Juicing!

By

Andrew Williams, Ph.D.

Version 1.1 Released 24th October 2013

PUBLISHED BY:

Juicing the Rainbow

Copyright © 2013

JuicingTheRainbow.com

Table of Contents

Medical Disclaimer

The information contained within this book is based upon research and personal experience of the author. The treatment outlined was devised by the author for his own personal use.

In no way must the information in this book be taken as medical advice. Restless Legs Syndrome (RLS), can be caused by serious medical conditions, and you need to see your doctor to make sure that your RLS is not a result of something more serious.

Before going on any form of alternative treatment (no matter how natural), you MUST consult your own doctor first, and discuss it with them.

If you decide to follow my own treatment plan, you do so at your own risk.

Juicing for Restless Leg Syndrome
Copyright © 2013

JuicingTheRainbow.com

Restless Legs Syndrome (RLS)

Since you are reading this, I assume that you suffer, or have suffered from this unpleasant condition, probably being kept awake at night as a consequence? I began to research restless legs syndrome when my wife was expecting our first baby. She suffered from it a lot during her pregnancy. Funnily enough, this was also the time that I too suffered from the sensations. Sympathy pains perhaps? I'm not sure.

I've heard a lot of different descriptions of how it feels during a "restless legs attack". These varying accounts may indicate that there are several causes to RLS, which would explain why each sufferer experiences something a little different. One thing's for sure; a lot more medical research needs to be done before we can fully understand the root causes of this condition.

To me, RLS felt like ants were crawling up the veins and arteries inside my legs. It was an incredibly unpleasant feeling of "energy" and sometimes had me jumping out of bed and running around on the spot. That would alleviate the problem while I was moving, but as soon as I stopped and lay down again, the "energy" would return.

My symptoms were very similar to some of the criteria that medical researchers use in the diagnosis of restless leg syndrome. These include:

1. Unpleasant feelings in the legs. If you have talked to your doctor about this, they might use words like Paresthesia or Dysesthesia. Don't panic if you hear terms like these. They simply mean sensations, with the latter word emphasising the unpleasantness of the sensation.

2. "Motor restlessness" which means the neurons that control the movement of your muscles are active (this can be voluntary movement as well as involuntary). Motor restlessness is characterised by an irresistible urge to move about. It should be noted that motor restlessness in patients with Parkinson's disease can be mistakenly diagnosed as RLS. However, most cases of RLS are nothing to do with Parkinson's disease.

3. Symptoms are worse when resting, with temporary relief during activity.

4. Symptoms are worse later in the day.

My wife always raised her legs up with pillows to reduce the symptoms, but this didn't seem to do much for me. I needed to find a different solution.

After a lot of research, I found out that there are a number of things that can cause RLS, most of which can be fixed easily, naturally, and without need of expensive or potentially dangerous medication.

The first section of this book looks at the condition. I will discuss the various causes that we know about, and explain who is most susceptible to them, etc. I'll be referring to medical literature, but don't worry I will simplify it into a language that is easy to understand. I will also provide links to web pages where you can find more information if you want to. When you see a number in square brackets like this **[1]**, it refers to a web page which you can find at the end of that section in this book. Not all of these citations will lead to the full article since many require a subscription to access the data. In those cases, I will direct you to viewable abstracts of those papers.

In the second half of the book I will outline a simple nutritional plan that I developed for my own use and which cured my restless legs. It consists of nothing more than an easy to follow nutritional plan. While this worked for me and my wife, I cannot *promise* it will work for you, but I am hopeful that it will be of benefit to many people suffering from this awful condition.

So on that note, let's now get on with exploring this all natural solution.

What Is Restless Leg Syndrome (RLS)?

RLS is a condition where the sufferer has a strong urge to move their legs (and in some cases their arms too), in response to unpleasant sensations in the limbs. Movement can temporarily relieve the symptoms. These symptoms are usually worse at night when you are inactive, and can cause insomnia as a result.

Because of the lack of sleep in some sufferers of RLS, those affected can often be fidgety, tired, and irritable the day following a restless night. If the condition lasts for several days, it can cause fatigue and emotional problems, including depression.

Who Is Most Likely to Get RLS?

Studies suggest that as much as 10% of the US population [1] may suffer from RLS, though the severity of the condition varies a lot between individuals. It's not just restricted to adults either, as children can suffer from this too (with some evidence suggesting that RLS has a genetic component and can therefore be passed on from parent to child).

RLS is a lot more common in women, and this may give us a clue to one of the causes of the condition, since women menstruate and lose blood regularly during their reproductive years. This wouldn't explain all cases in women though, since RLS can affect women of any age, so we'll come back to this later.

Pregnant Women Are More Likely to Get RLS

As if being pregnant didn't give enough aches, pains, and discomfort as it is, the sad fact is that pregnant women are far more likely to suffer from RLS than non-pregnant women. Thankfully, these symptoms quickly subside once the birth is out the way [2]. This correlation was first seen in the 1940s.

In an Italian study of 600 pregnant women, just over one quarter of them experienced RLS. For many of them, this was their first ever encounter of the condition. Of those who suffered from RLS, nearly all of them reported having at least one case of RLS per week, but around 50% of the sufferers reported having three or more episodes per week. The condition occurred mostly in the third trimester, but the good news is that once the baby was born, the majority of these women stopped having problems with RLS within four weeks of giving birth.

One of the potential causes of RLS is low iron. However, when a woman gives birth, she loses a lot of blood (which has a lot of iron locked up in haemoglobin), and may not fully recover her iron stores for a few months after delivery. Yet despite this fact, quite soon after accouchement, most women report that they no longer suffer from RLS. Studies on iron levels in women also tend to confirm, in this case at least, that iron is not the problem.

One thing that does change a lot during pregnancy and birth though are the hormone levels. It's possible that these changing levels are at least partially responsible for RLS in pregnancy.

Genetics May Play a Role

It's been suggested that up to 50% of those who suffer from RLS have a family history of the condition. Because it's only 50%, this suggests that genetics is not involved in the other 50%. Therefore, it seems probable that environmental factors must be involved, and research seems to supports this.

We have to be careful not to always assume that genetics are involved simply because a problem is occurring in generations of the same family. For example, if a family has a history of obesity, is that genetics? Isn't it also possible that generations within that family are obese because they eat the same type of unhealthy greasy foods? If you grow up on fried fatty snacks and meals, the chances are that this is what you are accustomed to AND likely to cook for yourself and your own family in the future. Learning bad habits is nothing to do with genetics; it's to do with environment.

Having said that, there is evidence of a genetic link for RLS. A number of studies have identified specific genes in the human genome that are found in some sufferers of RLS [3, 4].

More research really needs to be done though in order to identify how these genes can increase the risk of getting the condition.

Vitamin and Mineral Deficiencies

Let's now look at the various vitamin and mineral deficiencies that have been suggested as causes for RLS.

Iron Deficiency?

There have been a number of studies which look at the brains of people who suffer from RLS. The research suggests that some brain cells in the substantia nigra (mid-region of the brain that produces a lot of the neurotransmitter dopamine), are extremely low in iron. The problem may be linked with a protein receptor on the cell membrane called transferrin, which binds and transports iron into the cells. These cells seem to have very few of those receptors, so iron transfer into the cells is limited. This means that even if the person **doesn't** have an iron deficiency, they could still get RLS, simply because this part of the brain could not transfer enough iron into these cells [5].

A few studies have linked RLS to deficiencies in not only iron, but also dopamine. Without normal levels of iron, dopamine cannot be regulated properly [6]. It's interesting then that a number of medications that increase dopamine levels, such as the drug levodopa (L-Dopa), also help to alleviate RLS in some cases.

NOTE: levodopa is used in the treatment of Parkinson's disease.

OK; MLS may be (at least partly), due to the lack of iron in certain cells of the brain. This does not mean that everyone who suffers from RLS has a problem with transporter proteins.

Another obvious reason these cells might have low iron levels is that the patient actually *is* deficient in iron. If there are low iron concentrations in the blood, then there is less iron available to be transported into the brain cells.

The points below help to explain why:

1. A number of people have relieved their RLS symptoms by taking iron supplements.

2. Menstruating women normally suffer from iron deficiency due to blood loss.

WARNING: Taking iron supplements is not recommended without first seeking the advice of your doctor. Some people suffer from a hereditary disease called hemochromatosis. Their body stores too much iron and this can be very dangerous. In addition, excess iron supplementation can cause a host of medical problems, from simple constipation and nausea, to more serious health conditions.

Magnesium Deficiency?

Magnesium plays a hugely important role in the normal healthy functioning of our bodies, and is particularly vital in helping us get to sleep quicker, and sleep deeper [7, 8, 9, 10].

Some estimates suggest that up to 80% of people in the US are deficient in magnesium. The problem is that the soils our crops grow in have been depleted by aggressive farming methods, and the nutrients used up by the crops just haven't been replaced [11]. This holds true for many minerals, not just magnesium. In her book "How to know if you are Magnesium Deficient: 75 percent of Americans Are" [12], Liz Lipski explains how bad this has got.

In the 1930s the Department of Agriculture found the zinc levels in an average carrot to be 20 mg. In the 1980s, the level in an average carrot was just 10mg. Estimates today suggest this figure may be as low as 2 mg. This example just highlights the growing nutritional battle our bodies face as they try to extract the vitamins and minerals we need from our food. If mineral depleted soils were not enough to cope with, we are also accustomed to eating heavily processed foods, and the problem with this is that food processing diminishes the nutrient content.

So what do we know about magnesium that relates to RLS?

Well, we know magnesium deficiency increases neuromuscular excitability. We also know that magnesium supplementation can improve the sleep patterns of people deficient in magnesium.

Calcium Deficiency?

There are reports that calcium supplements can help relieve RLS symptoms. I read the story of a woman who suffered from RLS and took "Tums" (indigestion tablets made from calcium carbonate which are a readily absorbed form of calcium), for her mild heartburn, only to find that her RLS symptoms disappeared. Her husband also suffered RLS and found Tums alleviated his problems as well [13].

This actually makes a lot of sense, since calcium is required at neuromuscular junctions when a muscle contracts.

Potassium Deficiency?

I discovered a number of people who claimed that potassium supplementation helped them with their RLS [14, 15]. Some took potassium supplement pills, while others ate bananas before bedtime. Together with sodium, potassium is one of the two major electrolytes in our body. Maintaining the correct levels of potassium in the body is vital for muscle tone and contractions. The kidneys help regulate potassium (and sodium) levels in the body.

A deficiency in potassium can lead to muscle weakness or spasms, and even full blown paralysis in severe cases.

Folic Acid Deficiency?

The link with folic acid and RLS comes from pregnant women [16]. During the latter stages of pregnancy, folic acid levels can drop. This third trimester is when pregnant women typically suffer from RLS. So could a deficiency in folic acid be causing RLS during pregnancy?

Folic acid (and other B vitamins) is directly related to nerve health. High concentrations of folic acid (also called folate) are found in the spinal column. A deficiency can cause some confusion during the transmission of nerve impulses from the brain to elsewhere in the body.

There are certainly reported cases where folic acid cured RLS [17, 18]. It has also been suggested that people suffering from genetic RLS may have unnaturally high folic acid requirements. If you suffer this form of RLS, then maybe folic acid supplementation can help to alleviate your symptoms.

Medical Conditions

While many people can relieve their RLS symptoms by addressing their vitamin and mineral deficiencies, there are more serious causes of RLS, and you should make sure your doctor has ruled these possibilities out first.

- Kidney disease / final stage Kidney failure

- Peripheral nerve damage

- Diabetes

- Parkinson's disease

Other Possible Reasons for RLS

Unfortunately for many people, the following three "drugs" may play a part in RLS:

1. Caffeine

2. Alcohol

3. Tobacco

NOTE: Even chocolate has been implicated in RLS; so if you are overdoing it with the brown stuff, then it's time to cut back.

Studies have shown that in people who are susceptible to RLS, the above substances may trigger it. Simply by removing these from your life can be enough to prevent RLS occurring in some people.

References

1. http://www.ninds.nih.gov/disorders/restless_legs/detail_restless_legs.htm

2. http://www.ncbi.nlm.nih.gov/pubmed/21504414

3. http://www.rls.org/Document.Doc?&id=392

4. http://www.rls.org/Document.Doc?&id=414

5. http://www.ninds.nih.gov/news_and_events/news_articles/news_article_rls_iron.htm

6. http://www.sleep-journal.com/article/S1389-9457(04)00024-3/abstract

7. http://content.karger.com/ProdukteDB/produkte.asp?doi=10.1159/000118988

8. http://academic.research.microsoft.com/Publication/48517134/magnesium-involvement-in-sleep-genetic-and-nutritional-models

9. http://www.springerlink.com/content/hrl701m0417x4m13

10. http://academic.research.microsoft.com/Publication/33590575/should-we-use-oral-magnesium-supplementation-to-improve-sleep-in-the-elderly

11. http://www.canadianlongevity.net/misc/mineral_depletion.php

12. http://askdrgottmd.com/restless-legs-syndrome-responds-to-calcium/

13. http://books.google.com/books?id=VBZN4qTE
TogC&printsec=frontcover&redir_esc=y#v=one
page&q&f=false

14. http://www.healthboards.com/boards/restles
s-leg-syndrome/829713-potassium.html

15. http://www.rlcure.com/potassium.html

16. http://online.liebertpub.com/doi/abs/10.108
9/152460901750269652

17. http://www.earthclinic.com/CURES/restless_
legs2.html

18. http://www.healthboards.com/boards/restles
s-leg-syndrome/359511-simple-cure-some-
rls.html

How Is RLS Treated by Doctors?

Doctors will often suggest a number of lifestyle changes as a way to treat cases of restless legs syndrome. These may include things like:

- Sticking to a strict sleep schedule by going to bed at the same time every night.

- Doing moderate levels of exercise during the day (though high levels can actually make RLS worse).

- Giving up caffeine, alcohol and tobacco.

- Losing weight.

- Trying meditation.

- Muscle stretching (calves & thighs).

- Showers where you run hot/cold water over the legs before bedtime.

- Acupuncture.

- Try diverting your attention to something else whenever you get an RLS attack.

On April 6th 2011, the FDA approved a new drug called Horizant to treat RLS [1]. These are slow release tablets that are taken once a day. The active ingredient is gabapentin enacarbil, a substance that was denied approval by the FDA in February 2010. The reason given was:

"A preclinical finding of pancreatic acinar cell tumours in rats was of sufficient concern to preclude approval at this time."

In other words, there were concerns over the possible links with cancer!

In the body, gabapentin enacarbil becomes gabapentin, a drug used to treat seizures in people with epilepsy [2, 3]. Side effects mentioned on the FDA website are:

"May cause drowsiness and dizziness and can impair a person's ability to drive or operate complex machinery."

Other Drugs That Are Used to Treat RLS

There are a number of different types of drugs that are used to treat RLS. We can classify the five types of drugs according to the way they act.

1. **Dopaminergic drugs** - increase the levels of dopamine in the brain. Side effects include nausea, vomiting, hallucinations, and even involuntary movements.

2. **Dopamine Agonists** - these mimic dopamine in the brain. Side effects include sleepiness which can be a bad thing during the day. Examples of this type of drug used to treat RLS include ropinirole, pramipexole, carbidopa/levodopa, and pergolide.

3. **Benzodiazepines** - these are sedatives. They don't try to fix the cause of your RLS, they just allow you to get some sleep, e.g. diazepam. I have taken this myself and usually woke up the next morning feeling like I had a hangover. The only upside is they did help me sleep.

4. **Opioids** - Opiates are addictive so these tend to be a last resort. An example is Methadone.

5. **Anticonvulsants** - like Horizant we mentioned earlier. The active ingredients are actually used to treat epilepsy, but they can help with RLS symptoms, e.g. carbamazepine.

Here is a list of the common drugs that have been used to treat RLS:

- Gabapentin enacarbil (Horizant)

- Ropinirole (Requip, Ropark, Adartrel) - dopamine agonist often used to treat Parkinsons.

- Pramipexole (Mirapex, Mirapexin, Sifrol) - dopamine agonist.

- Carbidopa (Lodosyn) - taken in combination with levodopa in the treatment of Parkinsons.

- Levodopa, also called L-DOPA (Bendopa, Dopar, Eldopar, Laradopa, Larodopa, Levopa). Levodopa (with carbidopa) is found in the following Sinemet, Parcopa, Atamet, Stalevo. Levodopa (with benserazide) is found in

Madopar & Prolopa. L-DOPA is a natural substance made in the brain. It is converted into dopamine. Remember earlier we said that dopamine cannot be regulated properly in the absence of sufficient iron.

- Carbamazepine - anticonvulsant and mood-stabilising drug.

- Pergolide - a dopamine receptor agonist.

Sedatives are also prescribed to help the patient get some sleep. These may include:

- Clonazepam (Klonopin)

- Triazolam (Halcion)

- Eszopiclone (Lunesta)

- Ramelteon (Rozerem)

- Temazepam (Restoril)

- Zaleplon (Sonata)

- Zolpidem (Ambien)

The problem with drugs (besides the side effects) is that not all of them will work for everyone. You really will need to discuss the options with your doctor if you decide to go down the drug route.

References

1. http://www.fda.gov/NewsEvents/Newsroom/PressAnnouncements/ucm250188.htm

2. http://www.bellaireneurology.com/seizure/epil_trt_neurontin.html

3. http://www.ncbi.nlm.nih.gov/pubmed/12867216

Nutritional Approach to Curing Restless Leg Syndrome

As you've seen, Restless Legs Syndrome can be caused by a number of serious health problems, including Parkinson's disease, diabetes, nerve damage, and kidney disease. If you suffer from RLS syndrome, you should go to your doctor to make sure that something more serious is not the root of your problem. If your doctor clears you of these, then there is a good chance that your RLS is caused by nutritional deficiencies, and may be relieved in the same way my wife and I cured our own symptoms by focused nutrition.

I've mentioned earlier that alcohol, tobacco, and caffeine can also contribute to RLS. Therefore, to get a good night's sleep, I recommend you give these up for a while (or permanently if you can).

Hemochromatosis: I need to mention one more thing before we get into the program, and this is serious. Go to your doctor and make sure your iron levels are normal. A small percentage of the population suffer from a genetic disorder called hemochromatosis. Sufferers of this have abnormally high levels of iron in their body, especially in the liver. Since this nutritional program looks to supplement those vitamins and minerals that contribute to RLS when deficient, we will be looking to include iron-rich vegetables in the diet. Needless to say this could be dangerous for someone with hemochromatosis.

Which Nutrients Do We Need to Boost?

As we've seen earlier in this book, fruit and vegetables don't have the levels of minerals in them that they use to. This, and the fact we eat so much processed food, is probably to blame for a lot of the conditions we suffer from today. For this reason, the nutritional plan that I am going to outline contains the main five nutrients that have been reported to cause RLS, but also a lot of additional vitamins and minerals. The five main ones we want to concentrate on are:

1. Magnesium

2. Iron

3. Folic acid

4. Potassium

5. Calcium

Since these nutrients are available in raw fruits & vegetables, I have drawn up a list of "superfoods" that are rich in these 5 nutrients. In addition, I looked into herbal teas that could help me fall asleep (more on this later).

22

Restless Legs Syndrome "Superfoods"

In this section I want to highlight what I call the superfoods when it comes to RLS. These are the foods that contain high levels of the 5 essential nutrients listed above.

Here's a list of what these Superfoods contain:

All 5 of the Nutrients:

✓ • **Spinach** - magnesium, folic acid, potassium, calcium, iron

4 of the 5 Nutrients:

✓ • **Broccoli** - magnesium, iron, folic acid, potassium, calcium

• **Carrots** - magnesium, iron, potassium, calcium

• **Parsley** - magnesium, iron, potassium, calcium

3 of the 5 Nutrients:

• **Asparagus** - iron, folic acid, potassium

• **Beet greens** - magnesium, iron, calcium

• **Blackberries** - magnesium, iron, folic acid

• **Cabbage** - iron, potassium, folic acid

• **Cauliflower** - magnesium, iron, potassium

• **Celery** - magnesium, potassium, calcium

- **Dandelion greens** - magnesium, iron, calcium

2 of the 5 Nutrients:

- **Beets** - magnesium, iron
- **Oranges** - calcium, folic acid
- **Chard** - iron, potassium
- **Garlic** - magnesium, potassium
- **Kale** - folic acid, calcium
- **Watercress** - potassium, calcium

1 of the 5 Nutrients:

- **Pineapple** – iron
- **Radishes** – potassium
- **Romaine lettuce** – calcium
- **Strawberries** - iron
- **String beans** - calcium

Another good way to look at this information is by starting with the nutrient and then listing which fruit or vegetable they are rich in.

Here is that data:

- **Magnesium:** Beet greens, spinach, parsley, dandelion greens, garlic, blackberries, beets, broccoli, cauliflower, carrots, and celery.
- **Iron:** Parsley, dandelion greens, broccoli, spinach, cauliflower, strawberries, asparagus,

chard, blackberries, cabbage, beets with greens, carrots, and pineapple.

- **Folic acid:** Asparagus, spinach, kale, broccoli, cabbage, oranges, and blackberries.

- **Potassium:** Parsley, chard, garlic, spinach, broccoli, carrots, celery, radishes, cauliflower, watercress, asparagus, and cabbage.

- **Calcium:** Kale, parsley, dandelion greens, watercress, beet greens, broccoli, spinach, romaine lettuce, string beans, oranges, celery, and carrots.

OK, so we know which foods supply the essential vitamins and minerals we need. The idea is to eat a range of fresh produce which, as a whole, will provide your body with enough of each element.

You can do this one of two ways:

1. Eat the fruit and vegetables, preferably raw.

2. Juice those fruit and vegetables.

When I was treating my own RLS, I mainly concentrated on juicing for my nutrients. The reason for emphasising juicing was simply that I could "drink" more fruit & veg than I could comfortably eat. This was important, bearing in mind the lower levels of minerals in fresh produce nowadays.

Think about that for a minute.

There is a limit to the amount you can physically eat. You might be able to consume five carrots and half a head of broccoli, but you'd probably end up full and feeling a little uncomfortable. Yet I am sure I could juice those five carrots and half a head of broccoli, PLUS one beet, two oranges, a few leaves of chard, etc., and still end up with a drink that I could consume in one sitting.

What does this mean?

Well, it means you can get MORE of the vitamins and minerals by juicing than you can by just eating the produce.

NOTE: A lot of people wrongly state that by juicing you remove all the pulp. This was not the case with any juicer I tried. The only way you'd remove the pulp would be by sieving the juice after it's been made. Freshly made "unsieved" juice contains plenty of pulp (fibre), and the benefits associated with it.

In the next section of this book I will outline my own, personal plan.

If you DO NOT suffer from any of the medical problems listed above, then my proposal should be safe for you as well. However, **do consult your own doctor** and ask their advice before starting *any* nutritional program, including this one.

How I Cured My RLS - Nutritional Pla

Dietary Changes

I don't smoke, so this was not something I had to consider, but if you do, now is as good a time as any to give up.

My dietary changes involved a three-pronged attack.

1. Give It Up!

For a couple of weeks, while I was on my juicing plan, I gave up:

- Alcohol

- Caffeine (tea & coffee, plus soft drink containing caffeine)

2. Supplementing the Diet

One thing I added to my daily diet was raw foods chosen from the superfoods listed earlier. Here are the guidelines I followed:

> • Have a salad with at least one meal per day, using spinach (and dandelion greens if you can get them) instead of lettuce. Add in some grated carrots and a little chopped parsley (leave this out if you are pregnant). That is the basis of the salad. Feel free to include any other fruits or vegetables (even those that

27

are not on the superfood list) to make it taste to your liking. Make any type of dressing you like, but consider adding in a little crushed garlic into it.

• Chop up some carrots, cauliflower and celery, and leave them in the fridge. If you get hungry during the day, THESE are your snack foods. You can also eat bananas for snacks, as these provide a good source of potassium, magnesium, and folates, as well as other nutritionally important vitamins.

• If you can, find herbal teas that have any of the following in them: chamomile, valerian root, or passion flower. Drink your herbal before you go to bed. Of the three, valerian is probably the strongest sedative and **you should consult your doctor before taking any kind of natural tranquiliser**, especially if you are on other medications. Also, **if you are pregnant**, these are probably best avoided unless your doctor says it is OK.

In addition to the above, I supplemented my nutrition with fresh juice which I made in the mornings. I'd prepare about a litre of juice, and have a large glass straight away, and then sip the rest at different times throughout the day.

Let's look at the types of juice you can make.

3. Juicing

A lot of people like to have recipes to juice. I have always taken a different approach to juicing. What I do is look in my fridge or store cupboard, and pick up whatever I have available. It's a mix and match approach that works well for me. I guess that after a certain while you begin to know what flavours will work, and those that won't.

When juicing for specific vitamins and minerals, you can still take this mix and match approach, but your choice of fruit and vegetables is guided by the superfoods that contain the specific nutrients. You can add in other ingredients which are not on the superfood list, but the basis of your juice should be made with the superfoods.

I will give you some specific recipes in a moment, for those of you who would like step by step instructions. However, for those who want to try a mix-and-match approach, there are a few of guidelines that may help your juices taste better.

IMPORTANT FOR JUICERS: Make sure you thoroughly wash all fruit and vegetables before juicing. For oranges and lemons, remove the skin (white pith is OK). If you use apples, remove the pips.

Mix & Match Juicing Tips for the More Adventurous Juicer

Some vegetables have a very strong flavour that can overpower the juice and make it unpleasant to drink. These include:

- Watercress

- Garlic

- Beets (have a strong earthy flavour that some people don't like)

- Celery (especially if it's acutely green)

- Radishes

When you make a juice, go lightly on the above ingredients unless you know you like those strong flavours in your juice.

There are several items you can add that help neutralise strong tastes in your juices. These include:

- Oranges

- Carrots

- Berries

- Pineapple

- Cucumber (not a great source of the vitamins and minerals we need, but a good overall vegetable to use in your juices).

Recommended Mix-and-match "recipe"

I used a common base when making my juices to ensure I got the absolute best superfoods into them. These would provide the levels of nutrients I needed.

Juice Base:

- **A big handful of spinach.** Note: If you have a centrifugal juicer, you may not get much juice out of these. In that case, save your spinach for your daily salad (and buy baby spinach leaves as they are tenderer which makes them ideal for salads). If you have a masticating juicer (single or dual gear), then spinach can be juiced a lot more efficiently. For details on juicers, see my Best Juicer for Beginners article.

- **Five carrots**

- **A small handful of parsley.** IMPORTANT: If you are pregnant, do not use parsley on salad or in juice, as it can be toxic at high levels. For everyone else, don't go above a small handful a day. Again, if you are using a centrifugal juicer, save the parsley for your salads, as centrifugal juicers are not very efficient at extracting the juice from fine leaves. If you are using a masticating juicer, then add the parsley to your mix.

- **Two good fist sized florets of broccoli.**

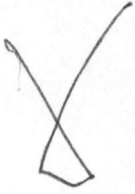

Put the spinach, carrots, parsley, and broccoli in your juicer. Then add in whatever superfoods you like. You can add in any fruit or vegetables that are not on the superfood list as well. This will prevent you from getting bored with your juices.

You should be aiming to make around one litre of juice every day. You can drink it all in one go, or drink half of it to begin with, and sip the rest during the day. Just remember to keep the leftover in the fridge.

If you want to add extra volume to your juice, oranges are excellent, as is cucumber, watermelon, and any other juicy fruit.

Juicing Recipes for the Less Adventurous

Before you start juicing, make sure the produce is well washed to remove any chemicals that might have been used in the production process.

For those of you who prefer to follow juice recipes, I have included five different ones below. I recommend you drink 2-3 DIFFERENT juices a day from this list, and for a period of 5-7 days (try to have all five juices over a two day period).

You should also be supplementing your diet as mentioned in the "Dietary Changes" section.

While each of these juices focuses on one main nutrient, the recipes do include most, if not all, of the required five nutrients we are trying to boost.

NOTE: If you need to "sweeten" a juice, add in an orange or two (peel removed), and/or a few carrots (washed but not peeled). These can help to make most juices taste better.

Recipe #1 - Magnesium Booster

- 6 carrots - washed but not peeled.

- 2 sticks of celery

- 1 beet with the greens.

- 2 fist-sized heads of broccoli

- One orange (skin removed but white pith is OK).

Recipe #2 - Iron Booster

- 2 fist-sized florets of broccoli
- 2 fist-sized florets of cauliflower
- 2 carrots
- Half a small pineapple (skin removed).
- 5 strawberries

Recipe #3 - Folic Acid Booster

- 2 fist-sized florets of broccoli
- One quarter of a small green cabbage.
- 3 oranges (peeled but white pitch is OK).
- 10 strawberries

Once the juice has been extracted, you can drink it as it is, or for an extra folic acid boost, whiz it up in a blender with half a small papaya, which will turn it into a smoothie.

Recipe #4 - Potassium Booster

- 5 Swiss chard leaves
- A small handful of parsley (if you are pregnant, leave this one out).
- 2 florets of broccoli
- 5 carrots
- 3 sticks of celery

Recipe #5 - Calcium booster

- 5 kale leaves
- A handful of dandelion leaves if available
- 2 florets of broccoli
- 2 oranges, peel removed (white pith is OK)
- 2 sticks of celery
- 2 carrots

If you find an ingredient you really don't like the taste of, just substitute it with one of the other superfoods that contains the same nutrient. You can also adjust ingredient portions if you find the recipes make too much or too little juice with your juicer.

How Long Before RLS Is Gone?

Obviously everyone is different - that includes the severity of the problem and the root cause of the condition.

I stayed on this program for about a week, but my RLS symptoms were gone within just two days of starting. I obviously cannot promise you the same rapid relief for the reasons mentioned above.

You might find that your RLS disappears while on the program, but returns once you come off it. If that happens, I would suggest that some of the dietary changes you made should become permanent dietary changes, especially the consumption of more raw fruit and vegetables (particularly dark green vegetables like spinach, kale, parsley, and chard).

Since I completed this program, I have started regular juicing and try to incorporate these superfoods into my daily juice program. For example, I still use baby spinach in salads instead of lettuce, and thankfully my RLS has never returned. In addition to this, I feel younger, rarely get sick, and have a lot more energy than I use to have. Needless to say that juicing has become a way of life for me.

I hope this program will also help you get rid of your RLS!

If you enjoyed this book, then please consider leaving a review on Amazon.

This is my first book in a "Juicing for.." series.

You can find my other Kindle books here:
http://JuicingTheRainbow.com/kindle

And you can contact me through my website at:

JuicingTheRainbow.com

10180506R00027

Printed in Great Britain
by Amazon.co.uk, Ltd.,
Marston Gate.